God Wants You Healed
By Dr. Marilyn S. Murphree

Preface 5/

Chapter 1 The Prayer of Faith 6/

Chapter 2 Binding, Rebuking, and Loosing 10/

Chapter 3 Speak to the Mountain 14/

Chapter 4 The Laying on of Hands and Anointing with Oil 19/

Chapter 5 Why Try to Get it When You Have Already Got It 21/

Chapter 6 Who Cares? 24/

Chapter 7. In the Name of Jesus 26/

Chapter 8 God Wants you Well 30/

Chapter 9 Count Those Things that Be Not as Though they Were 34/

Chapter 10   Like a Tree Planted by the Water   38/

Chapter 11 Prayer Cloths   42/

Chapter 12 The Blood of Jesus 45/

Chapter 13 The Power of Agreement   50/

Chapter 14 The Power of Praise 54/

Chapter 15 Imparting the Life of Jesus   58/

Chapter 16 When God Answered   61/

Chapter 17 The Strongman   65/

Chapter 18 Speedy Healing   69/

Chapter 19 Praying in the Spirit   74/

Chapter 20 The Healing Power   78/

Preface

I did not plan to write another book on healing. What more could be said? I had been struggling for almost five years to fully recover from a stroke. I could not walk at all. After months of therapy, I was able to walk but not like I had before the stroke. In spite of much prayer and others praying for me, I felt I was not making progress like I should be. Someone said, "If you are not making any progress on your healing, ask the Lord for a fresh word from Him."

I asked the Lord for a fresh word but nothing came to mind, but days later a thought occurred and I wrote it down. This was what came to mind.

"Don't keep asking for the same things over and over again." It was as if the Lord said, "Excuse me, I heard you the first time."

Later another thought came to mind. It was, "Agree with God. Don't disagree with what He says. When He says, "I am the Lord that healeth you," don't say, "No, Sir, I am still sick and I still hurt."

I wrote this book to help me to get some additional insights on healing, and I did. I hope it will give you some as well. Although it is my fourth book on healing, I have continued to grow in my understanding that God wants us to be healed.

Chapter 1
The Prayer of Faith

James 5:15, "And the prayer of faith shall save the sick, and the Lord shall raise him up; and if he have committed sins, they shall be forgiven him."

The prayer for healing is a specific kind of prayer. It is not a begging type of prayer or and if it be Thy will kind of prayer. The verse in James clearly states that the prayer of faith shall save the sick and the Lord will raise him up. It is a clear statement of confidence that the Lord will indeed do something about the problem. Not maybe in His good old time, but He will raise the sick person up. We know of people who say they are praying for you. What does it mean when someone says, "I am praying for you every day, but nothing happens?" You don't get better and nothing happens? There might be a lot of things taking place, and the healing is blocked for some reason. Maybe it is a prayer just containing empty words or filled with doubt and unbelief. Maybe the person praying doesn't really believe in healing for today. Is the prayer an effective one or just words?

Another clue is, "the effectual fervent prayer of a righteous man availeth much" (James 5:15). The prayer has to be more than a few words on a piece of paper. There has to be some life in the words. The word *fervent* is contained here. It is a prayer that means business and expects something to happen.

After the prayer for a sick man, the pastor asks, "Bill, what are you going to do tomorrow?" to which he replied, "Why pastor, I'm going to be right here sick in bed."

An effectual fervent prayer has a different expectation than that. After the Amen one would hope that a person would see a change taking place. An expectation should be there once the prayer of faith is spoken. Perhaps the person has been prayed for many times in the past and did not see results. It is true this may have happened and disappointment occurred. Scripture says, "Cast not therefore away your confidence which has great recompense of reward" (Hebrews 10:35). That is saying, "Hold on to your confidence that the answer is on the way." Can you hang on a little bit longer when the answer doesn't come immediately? The prayer of faith is different from a dry lifeless prayer of *maybe* it will happen. Not the prayer if I wonder if it will happen or maybe it won't happen today or maybe God won't do it for me. That is not the prayer of faith. What is faith anyway? Scripture says,

"Faith is the substance of things hoped for, the evidence of things not seen" (Hebrews 11:1). A further explanation is that faith is the confidence that what we hope for will actually happen (Hebrews 11:1 NIV). Or faith is the assurance of things hoped for (English Standard Version).

The prayer of faith will save the sick and God will raise him up. God will indeed do it. God is not a man that He should lie. Another scripture says, "Thy Word is truth" (John 17:17). The devil puts a lot of pressure on us to just give up after it has not happened in a reasonable amount of time. There is not a certain time limit put on the promises of God. The length of time might vary from person to person or problem to problem. Do we have to have a specific time limit put on answers? The main thing is to get the problem resolved and the answer to come. "Thy Word Oh Lord is settled in heaven" (Psalm 119:89).

I Peter 1:25 says, "But the Word of the Lord endures forever."

The prayer of faith is a prayer of total confidence and assurance that the answer is on the way. Scripture says, "Ask and it shall be given, seek and ye shall find, knock and it shall be opened to you" (Matthew 7:7-8). It does not say *maybe some day*. It says, "Ask, and it shall be given." Are you asking for something that is within your right to ask for are you asking amiss? Some prayers may need to be reframed. Find some scriptures to stand on that clearly states that it is within God's will for you. Is healing a promise for you?

By his stripes ye *are* healed.

By his stripes ye *were* healed.

I am the Lord that healeth thee.

I will restore health to you and heal you of all your wounds.

Beloved I wish above all things that ye may prosper and be in health even as thy soul prospers.

He sent his word and healed them.

The effectual fervent prayer based on our rights avails much. Ask. Go ahead and ask for what you need standing on the promises of God. He said that healing is the children's bread. Take *your* healing for whatever it is you need.

I need healing. So I am asking based on Your Word that is truth. Thy Word O Lord is truth. I take the healing that has been provided for me on the cross. I take it by faith and believe in your Word that it is there for me. By his stripes I am healed.

Chapter 2
Binding, Rebuking, and Loosing

I rebuke all pain in the Name of Jesus, and I command it to get out of my body right now. I rebuke all spirits of infirmity, nerve disorder, lung damage in the name of Jesus. Thank you Jesus.

Jesus has given us authority to bind and rebuke the works of the devil and expect it to happen no matter how overwhelming the situation seems to us. We are to loose the good things into our life as well. Driving Satan back with a stern rebuke is not enough to make him keep his distance. He always tries to sneak up on us again, and we need to go after him through the tools Jesus gave us for defeating him. Jesus spoke sharply to Satan in scripture and didn't allow him to get a foothold. As Christians we are reminded not to give Satan a foothold when he comes lurking around in our weakest moments. Ephesians 4:27 NIV says, "And do not give the devil a foothold." Do not pray a passive prayer but aggressively go after him by rebuking him when he comes to steal from you. Stealing is just the first step. He wants to not only steal from you but to kill and to completely destroy you. It doesn't have to be that way. "We overcome by the blood of the lamb and the word of our testimony" (Revelation 12:11). We often think that things happen automatically, but they don't. We have to take our rights that have been provided. We must know what they are and speak out aggressively in faith. When pain comes to our body, don't passively say, "Well, I am getting older, and it is to be expected." Say, "No, I am overcoming by the blood of the Lamb and the word of my testimony. I am healed by His stripes. I will not tolerate this pain any more. I will rebuke it and bind it in the Name of Jesus. And I will loose the healing that is rightfully mine. I cover myself with the blood of the Lamb and the blood of Jesus has power to do the work. The old song goes, "Oh, the blood of Jesus has never lost its power."

I will take authority over sickness and disease not in my own strength but through the Name of Jesus our Lord and Savior. We miss out because we think that this is the way things have to be. Who says? It is the devil who deceives us with lies and tells us that healing doesn't happen in the 21st century. Jesus, however, is "the same Yesterday today and forever" (Hebrews 13:8). He healed terminal disease back then. He is perfectly able to do it today as well, but we let people talk us out of what is rightfully ours. Christian friends can be filled with doubt even more so than unbelievers and slip it to us in very few words and cause us to agree with them. Of course we don't want to look foolish to believe something so preposterous now do we? But you know in your heart that you want to be well again. Scripture says to "resist the devil (in whatever form he comes) and he will flee from you." It may take more than one time to resist him until you see the results you are after. Learn to guard your heart against what people tell you. The Word of God is final authority. Scripture says, "Thy Word, O Lord, is settled in heaven" (Psalm 119:89), and "Thy Word is Truth" (John 17:17). It is not the doubt and unbelief of friends and relatives or authority figures that is truth. Scripture says, "Ye shall know the truth and the truth shall set you free" (John 8:32).

When you are coming against the work of the enemy, it is better to speak God's Word out loud to him rather than silently in your mind. Speak it out loud and in no uncertain terms. "I bind you Satan in the Name of Jesus and rebuke the pain in my body at the Source." Don't just deal with the symptoms. The pain might not be coming from where it hurts. The parts of the body are intertwined—the nerves travel all over and can cause pain that a person would not suspect it coming from. Say, "I bind this pain at the source. I speak to pain and say, ""Pain leave my body now. You have no right to stay here another minute. Pain I rebuke you and the enemy who brought it."

Scripture says, "Ask and ye shall receive" (John 16:24). You receive at the time you ask by faith. The pain may not leave immediately and this could very easily cause you to be discouraged and say "It's no use. I give up." That's what the devil wants you to do. He wants you to make your pain your friend and take it everywhere you go and tell all your friends what an awful time you're having. Don't be succored in by that. You are not after sympathy. You are after wellness.

"I bind and rebuke this pain at the root in the Name of Jesus the same yesterday, today, and forever. I loose the healing I need right now and receive it today. Thank you Jesus. I am overcoming by the blood of the Lamb and the word of my Testimony." Praise the Lord!

Chapter 3

Speak to the Mountain

I speak to the mountain!

Don't ask God to speak to the mountain for you. He told you to say to the mountain, "Be thou removed and be cast into the sea." Mountain of pain in my hands I speak to you and say be thou removed from my body from the root source whether it is coming from my shoulder or wherever it is coming from and be thou removed and cast into the sea. Pain be out of my body. You have no right to be here because by his stripes I am healed. The power of God is in me to drive out sickness and disease. By his stripes I was already healed. Pain you can't stay in my body because I am healed. Legs be healed in the Name of Jesus. I call forth the healing power of God into my legs and hands and neck. I call forth the healing power of Jesus wherever it is in my my body that needs healing.

Be specific about speaking it.

Once and for all be thou removed, not just tolerated or made manageable. I speak to the pain in an assertive way and say, "You can't stay in my body. God in the Name of Jesus."

When you pray, be specific. Pin point the problem that is troubling you. Call it out. I say, "Pain I take authority over you in the Name of Jesus and say, "I drive you out now. Be thou removed and be thou cast into the sea and don't return." One woman said, "And devil don't return for 24 hours," but say, "go and don't return at all. Be gone. I am done with you! And mean it. Be gone in the Name of Jesus." Instead of taking a couple aspirins say, "Headache be gone in the Name of Jesus. I take authority over you now. I speak with the delegated authority of Jesus. Along with the speaking, I believe it will happen." Matthew 28:14 says, "All authority in heaven and in earth has been given to me."

John 16:23 backs this up by saying, "Whatever ye ask of the Father in my Name, I will give it unto you."

Our words have a powerful effect on the mountains that loom high before us. We think we can't climb them or tunnel through them or go around them, but our words spoken in the name of Jesus can penetrate the insurmountable mountain. Do not be hesitant or fearful. Whatever you say—it will work if you say it.

Formulate words against your mountains. If you hesitate speaking those words out in faith, practice looking into a mirror and say those words aloud. "I speak to this pain in my hand in the Name of Jesus. Pain I command you to leave now in the name of Jesus. You cannot stay." What if nothing happens? Say it again and mean it. Scripture says, "Resist the devil and he will flee from you. Not maybe. He will. Our words must be spoken with faith that they will be effective against anything that the devil hurls at us.

Say with authority, "Be thou removed." Get out and don't return to harass me.

Once you have spoken to the problem, expect something to happen. Don't say, "I wonder if..." Start to immediately say, "Thank you Jesus for the answer. It is done. By His stripes I am healed. It's a "done deal." Start acting like you are a different person. Pick something you couldn't do before and try to do it even if you can't do it with record speed. Put one foot ahead of the other. Type with that bum hand. Do something out of the ordinary. Don't think you can do it? Make the attempt in faith. "I believe I can do it." Say this out loud. "I believe I can do it."

"I can do all things through Christ which strengtheneth me." What do you do if you outright fail?

You could reevaluate and try it again. Say, "I say pain go in the name of Jesus and try it again."

One scripture that tells us never to give up is, "And let us not be weary in well doing for in due season we shall reap if we faint not" (Galatians 6:9).

Hebrews 6:12 cautions us "not to be lazy but to imitate those who through faith and patience inherit what has been promised"(NIV). Patience may take a little while to see it happen or a long while. You have spoken to the problem to go and ordered it out of your body—you have believed that it will happen and you have looked in the mirror and spoken it assertively. You have tried to do something as a step of faith even if ever so slowly. Then you rest in the presence of God and let patience have her perfect work. James 1:4-8 says, "Let patience have her perfect work that ye may be perfect and entire wanting nothing."

The NIV says, "Let perseverance finish its work so that you may be mature and complete, not lacking anything."

The Good News Translation puts it this way. "Make sure that endurance carries you all the way without failing, so that you may be perfect and complete, lacking nothing." Be sure to keep on going until you get to the finish line where the answer has arrived and is manifest in your body.

Do more than speak to the problem in the beginning. Move through faith and patience until you get to the finish line and see the results you are looking for

Praise the Lord! I've got it!

Chapter 4
The Laying On of Hands and the Anointing With Oil

The laying on of hands is both a symbolic and formal method of invoking the Holy Spirit in various types of services. For one, in prayer for healing where there is also the anointing with oil. James 5:14-16 with reference to the laying on of hands and healing scripture asks the question, "Is there any sick among you?" And then gives an answer about what to do. "Call for the elders of the church and let them pray over him, anointing him with oil in the name of the Lord and the prayer of faith shall save the sick and the Lord shall raise him up: and if he have committed sins they shall be forgiven him."

The sense of touch is one Jesus used in many cases when a person came for healing. Often he would merely lay hands on the person and say, "Be healed." Luke 5:13-15 ERV Jesus said, "I want to heal you. Be healed!" Then he touched the man and immediately the leprosy disappeared." Luke 13:10-17 NLT "when Jesus saw her, he called her over and said, "Dear woman, you are healed of your sickness! Than he touched her, and instantly she could stand straight." Touch appeared be the point of contact between the person and Jesus and power was transferred to bring about the healing. Jesus did not heal by just one method. It depended on the person and the situation. In one case scripture said, "He sent his word and healed them" (Psalm 107:20). And he delivered them from their destruction.

Chapter 5
Why Try to Get it When You Have Already Got it?

"Excuse Me! I heard you the first time."

"Ask and ye shall receive, seek and ye shall find, knock and it shall be opened unto you" (John 16:24).The first thing in this scripture was to ask, but it does not say to ask the same thing over and over every day and you will receive but simply to ask.   Too many days go by and we ask the same thing over and over again with no results. Months go by and we are still asking the same prayer over and sometimes the years slip by and we are still asking the same thing over and over.

This is when God says, "Excuse me, but I heard you the first time. It is now time to get out of the asking stage and get on to the receiving stage. Connected to the asking is the receiving. Maybe it is immediate and maybe it is not. But it says the receiving follows the asking. Ask and you shall receive.

Scripture says, "with his stripes ye are healed" (Isaiah 53:5)). In the New Testament it says, "by whose stripes ye were healed (I Peter 2:24).   This New Testament scripture indicates that your healing has already taken place and that your struggle is not trying to get it because you already have it as a part of Jesus' work on the cross. You don't have to try to get it because you've already got it, but it hasn't manifest itself in your body yet. You bring it into manifestation by thanking the Lord that He has already done it and that it is yours now by faith. Your faith shall make you whole. Praise and thanksgiving take us to the next stage. Do not keep asking for the same thing over and over again as if you are begging God to cause Him to give it to you. God wants you well. He told us this in III John. "Beloved I wish above all things that ye prosper and be in health even as your soul prospers." Sometimes we think God is holding out on us but Psalm 84:11 says, "No good thing will he withhold from them that walk uprightly." If He is wanting us to be well, that is not a sign for us to ask the same thing over repeatedly day after day. He assures us, "I am the Lord that healeth thee" (Exodus 24:26).

We must call it forth from our spirit into our body. Thank God I am healed because the Word says so and "thy word O Lord is settled in heaven" (Psalm 119:89). The word settled give us the assurance and makes a demand on what is promised to us. We can stand on the Word of God as true and that it will happen as we declare it. We can make the statement, "I am healed by his stripes and expect it to happen."

Continue to expect the answer is on the way in spite of things looking worse. The devil tries to throw you off track by making things look worse. He wants you to confess, "I am doing worse today than I was yesterday" and derail our faith. This is the time to put a zipper on our lips. Don't confess the negative thoughts by putting them into words for the enemy to run with. We have asked and we have received so don't accept anything less than that. "Ask and ye shall receive." Don't know the exact time the pain will actually leave your body but it will go as you release your faith and don't back down. You have already spoken to the pain to go—to be removed and cast into the sea and you have believed in your heart that it is so whether you see it yet or not. Speak the Word when in doubt. Speak it out loud. By his stripes I was healed and *if I was healed, I am healed right now*. The healing will manifest itself in my physical body and the pain will go. The wellness will come into being and my body will be whole. I have cast out the spirit of infirmity that has been making me weak. "They that wait upon the Lord shall renew their strength, they shall mount up on wings as eagles and they shall run and not be weary and walk and not faint (Isaiah 40:31).

Teach me Lord to wait.

Chapter 6
Who Cares?

"Lord, Carest thou not that we perish?"

Their confidence in Jesus was low at that point in the storm. They were convinced that He must not care about what happened to them. "Don't you care Lord?' they shouted. We often feel the same way when the wind and waves blow up around us threatening our very lives. Don't you care about the throbbing pain, Lord? Can't you do something about it?—right now?

Many of our emergency prayers seem to go unnoticed by the Lord, and we wonder if He indeed cares about what happens to us.

Scripture reminds us not to cast our confidence away. "Cast not therefore your confidence away which has great recompense of reward" (Hebrews 10:35). We have many uncertainties as well as the disciples about whether He will rescue us in time. Does He even know about our dilemmas? What's more, does He care about it? What if He lets me fail? What if he doesn't heal me? What if nothing can be done about my situation, and I perish? All of these thoughts frantically swirl around in our minds during the crises moments. The *what ifs* and the *maybes* sink us many times. Satan puts strong pressure on us not to believe and to conclude that the days of old are past. What can we do about these suggestions of Satan to work at tearing us down?

Jesus had the answer when he asked His disciples, "Don't you have any faith?" (Mark 4:40). I think his disciples were somewhat quiet when He asked that question.

Jesus is asking them, "Don't you have any faith in me that I can handle this problem?" Apparently it was obvious that they didn't. They thought they were going to drown and they let Jesus know that they didn't think He cared.

Jesus wanted them to work on their faith and not throw it away. That was their confidence in His ability to do something about the situation at hand. Would they have any more faith the next time a storm occurred? Will we have any more faith the next time a crisis comes on us suddenly? Don't know. We would hope so.

Chapter 7
In the Name of Jesus

Who do we pray to? Jesus, the Holy Spirit, the Virgin Mary, or to God the Father? Scripture gives us the model prayer when Matthew 6 begins, "Our Father which art in heaven, hallowed be thy Name." In another scripture Jesus told His disciples, "hitherto ye have asked nothing in My Name, ask and ye shall receive that your joy may be full" (John 16:24).

We are instructed to ask the Father in the name of Jesus. What is so important about this?

Philippians 2:9-11 tells us the importance of the Name of Jesus. "Wherefore God also hath highly exalted him and given him a Name which is above all names that at the Name of Jesus every knee should bow, of things in heaven and things in earth and that every tongue should confess that Jesus Christ is Lord to the glory of God the Father." Jesus told His disciples, "Whatsoever you ask the Father in my Name, he will give it to you" (John 16:23). Why ask in the name of Jesus? "Whatever you ask in my Name this will I do that the Father be glorified in the Son" (John 14:13). Why ask in the Name of Jesus? We know that the name of Jesus is effective because "All authority," Jesus said,

"In heaven and on earth has been given to me" (Matthew 28:18).

Jesus is Someone Whom God has put in charge of doing something about any problem. He has the ultimate authority to move mountains. Here is what many people don't know. We have been delegated this same authority.

"Behold I have given you authority over all the power of the enemy and you can walk on snakes and scorpions and crush them. Nothing shall by any means hurt you" (Luke 10:19). In Matthew 16:18 Jesus said, "The gates of hell shall not prevail." Every believer has power and authority to defeat Satan and all evil spirits.

Colossians 1:13 tells us, "who hath delivered us from the power of darkness, and hath translated us into the kingdom of his dear son." The word power is translated authority. You and I have been delivered from the authority of darkness and placed into God's kingdom and this world and the enemy have no authority over us. We have been delivered from it, but we must know that we have been. We must speak with our authority and walk in our authority. When Jesus appeared to His disciples after the resurrection, He delegated the authority to them. He told them, "Go ye into all the world and preach the gospel to every creature. "He that believeth and is baptized shall be saved; but he that believeth not shall be dammed. And those signs shall follow them that believe; In My Name shall they cast out devils; they shall speak with new tongues; they shall take up serpents, and if they drink any deadly thing it shall not hurt them; they shall lay hands on the sick and they shall recover" (Mark 16:15-18).

You must know your authority and accept it so that when you go to the throne of grace as mentioned in Hebrews 4:16 you will have no hesitation whatsoever. You have permission to go to God's throne boldly and ask. If you are not sure about your authority, how can you ask and see it done. In Christ we already have that authority. We need to believe it and walk in it. We must begin to take back what the devil has stolen from us— our health, our finances, our relationships, peace, and joy. The devil comes to steal, kill, and destroy. Don't let him. Everything the devil has stolen from you, you have the right to but it is your responsibility to take authority over the enemy and not allow him to steal from you.

Ephesians 1:21-23 says, "All things are under Jesus' feet."

When you speak the Name of Jesus the power behind the Name of Jesus is the power of the almighty God.

Jesus' Name can do anything He can do. He is totally unlimited. Begin operating in His Name. Lay hands on the sick and speak healing in the Name of Jesus.

Chapter 8
God Wants You Well

Why do people fight against healing? On one hand the parking lots at hospitals are filled. Doctor's appointments fill our calendars. People try the latest prescriptions, all kinds of supplements, therapies, and spend thousands of dollars to get well, but at the same time, they fight against being healed. Instead they say it may not be God's will to heal me or maybe this sickness has come on me to teach me something. Maybe Jesus just healed people back then to get the church started. God doesn't heal people today or at least it doesn't happen very often. That is why we have the medical profession today. When people read the Bible, they say it doesn't mean that in the 21st century. It's preposterous to think that God wants us well. You know that "time and chance" happens to us all. You know that when you get older you are going to experience pain and sickness and disease.

Who says? The devil puts on pressure to believe the world's philosophy. Times have changed, people say, and they let the devil convince us that this is gospel truth. We begin to buy into this philosophy when we take ownership for sickness and disease. Don't ever make sickness and disease your friend by saying, "My diabetes, my fibromyalgia, my high blood pressure—" on and on it goes where people take on ownership of all sorts of sickness. This is the devil's trap, the first step off getting you hooked on a downward path. Jesus has paid for our healing, but we invite pain and destruction into our bodies. People wake up hurting and go to bed hurting, and they think that it is just normal and to be expected. Oh yes, they would like to feel a little bit better or a whole lot better, but they tolerate pain because they think that this is the way things have to be. Healing is a part of what Jesus did on the cross for us, but we try to explain away what Jesus provided for us. It is not God's will for you to be sick and struggling day after day. Weeks go by, months and turning into years. We have to first of all change our thinking—God wants you well. We must decide not to tolerate sickness and disease because God has never told you that it has been done away with in our day.

Can we establish the fact that "by his stripes we are healed?" and "I am the Lord that healeth thee?"

We must not only believe that He is our healer but that He wants to make it happen for us. We say bind and rebuke the pain and cast out the spirit of infirmity, but we often let the devil slip back in on us. To the point where we couldn't retain the improvement. We cannot say, "Whatever will be will be" thinking that just maybe our answer will never happen. Just accept it. No, we don't have to accept it. We must continue on and don't ever give up on God. What needs to be changed will be changed as time goes by. The healing will come whether or not the healing comes instantly or gradually. The power of God is in me to drive out sickness and disease.

God has already done His part. We are not waiting on God. He put the same power that He put into Jesus into me. God is not holding out on us.

"Thank you God, I speak to the problem. I don't speak to God about the problem. I just rebuke the things that try to come on me. I am healed in the Name of Jesus."

If the symptoms come back, don't tolerate it by backing down and saying, "Maybe God doesn't want to do it for me."

"No, we have already decided that God wants us well—Beloved I wish above all else..." Are we going to back down on what scripture says?

Today we have an opportunity to receive and to be blessed. Jesus is here to save you, heal you, prosper you and deliver you from the oppression of the devil. We can make a decision to make sickness our friend and welcome into our life or in no way tolerate it. I choose to believe that what Jesus said is what He truly meant for us to have. We have to believe that what He said was true and quit trying to explain healing away for today. It is for us today.

Today I receive what You have for me. I am healed by His stripes. Praise God!

Chapter 9

Count Those Things That Be not as Though They Were

How do we move on from the problem to the answer? We quit talking about the problem and all the symptoms. Quit talking about the pain. You are moving out of pain because the power of God is in you to drive out sickness and disease. The blood of Jesus has freed you from the curse and you are no longer living in pain. Jesus has broken the yoke, but you have to recognize that you are now free in Christ and His work on the cross. What do you do when the pain hasn't left yet? Do like Abraham did. He counted those things that were not [yet] as though they were [now]. Build a vision of wellness right now. I'm healed by his stripes. Shift gears to move out of the pain and problems into the now. I am already healed. My body just doesn't know it yet, but I am moving in that direction. If I am already healed by his stripes and counting it so, how would I act? How would I be different? I thought about this for quite a while. For one thing I wouldn't be talking about my sickness all the time. If you are well, you don't talk sickness and disease. You wouldn't be telling all your friends about your friend the sickness. Eliminate *my* from your vocabulary. Don't say any more my fibromyalgia, or my diabetes, or *my* whatever it is. You do not take ownership for any of these sicknesses and diseases. That day is past and you are living in wellness today. You can now begin to do things you couldn't do before even if you have to take baby steps. You might not be there yet but at least you have started. Philippians 1:6 says, "Being confident of this very thing, that He which hath begun a good work in you will perform it until the day of Christ Jesus." The scripture doesn't say how quickly He will perform it or complete it or finish it. In His time He will get it done. If healing is what you need, He will unfold wellness. You must believe that wellness is on the way and say, "When I am well' "not if I ever get well." Visualize yourself as a well person now. Count those things that be not [yet] as though they were [already]. Program your mind to think like Abraham did. Post a picture of yourself when you looked your best and could do the things you wanted to do. Then say faith building words such as, "I can do all things thorough Christ which strengtheneth me" (Philippians 4:13). Practice doing a new thing today that you struggled to do last week. Repeat faith building scriptures such as Isaiah 58:8 NIV, "Then your light will break forth like the dawn, and your healing will quickly appear, then your righteousness will go before you and the glory of the Lord will be your rear guard."

Expect the blessing of the Lord to be upon you. Sickness is not a blessing. Speak positive things associated with the blessings of God. Galatians 3:14-20 talks about the blessing of Abraham and that it might come on the Gentiles through Jesus Christ that we might receive the promise of the Spirit through faith.

Verse 29 says, "And if ye be Christ's, then are ye Abraham's seed, and heirs, according to the promise." We can follow the pattern of Abraham when he counted those things that be not [yet] as though they are [now].

What are the "be nots" in your life that plague you day after day? A health problem that lingers on and on or a financial problem that nips at your heels never letting go? A sense of depression that weighs you down and never lifts?

Recovering from something that has hit us out of the blue can be a "be not" because it can linger from one week to the next no matter what it seems we do to alleviate the problem. One such thing is recovering from a stroke or a heart attack or cancer with all of the accompanying fears. Will I ever get well? Will God do it for me? Will He do it today or has the days of healing passed? Are the days of prosperity over? Will I ever have peace in my life? Our "be nots" could be any number of things, but he looked on them with eyes of a vision for the future. Abraham counted those things that "be not" as though they were [now] and couldn't accept anything less than that. Begin to look at your be nots like Abraham and say, "I count the thing that is bugging me day after day as though it were a prayer answered. I counted those things that be not as though they were today. It's no sweat to God. All things are possible to him that believeth. Thank you God.

Chapter 10
Like a Tree planted by the Water

"Old age ain't no place for sissies" is a saying on my coffee mug. Advancing years brings a variety of aches and pains that would like to take over in our body and bring along a feeling of discouragement and depression if we let it. As birthdays come and go we often try to make a joke of them and say, "I'm over the hill now" or we give someone a bunch of black balloons for their birthday or a rear view mirror. We have many scriptures that tell us that we should be optimistic about every stage of our life. We have heard the saying, "When things get tough, the tough get going." Healing does not cease just because we have reached a certain number of years in our lives. The verse, "I am the Lord that healeth you" doesn't one day expire and you wake up finding that the Lord has forsaken you. In the Psalms David cried out to the Lord, "Do not discard me in my old age, do not forsake me when my strength is gone" (Psalm 71:9). Isaiah 46:4 NIV has an answer for us, "Even in your old age and gray hair, I am he who will sustain thee. I have made you and I will carry you;

and will sustain you; and rescue you." We will not "just exist" as we age but we can continue to be a fruitful person. Psalm 92:14 tells us, "In old age they will still bear fruit." The verse goes on to say even in your old age I will be the same. Well, doesn't scripture say, "Jesus Christ the same yesterday today and forever?" David looks back to days past and says, "O God, you have taught me from my youth, and to this day I declare your wondrous works" (Psalm 71:17 NKJV).

"I will hope continually and will praise you yet more and more" (Psalm 71:14).

Because of God's faithfulness throughout all of life's stages, we will continue to hope in him and praise him.

Scripture says the Lord inhabits the praise of his people. He lives right in the middle of our praises. Let us be assured that He indeed does hear us when we call out to him just like David did. I John 5:15 NIV says, "And if we know He hears us,--whatever we ask—we know that we have what we asked of Him." Other translations say we already have it. So praise and thanksgiving right now is appropriate.

Not only will the Lord sustain us and keep us productive but scripture likens us to a tree that is planted by the water—not a tree that just sprang up out of nowhere but a tree that is cared for and tended regularly and this tree shall stay fresh and green and bear fruit.

Do you feel old and unfruitful? Be encouraged God still has fruitful ministry for you to do. Psalm 71:16 says, "I will go in the strength of the Lord God." I will put one foot ahead of the other and keep going for He sustains me.

What is the key to bearing fruit now you know that it is possible? The key is found in John 15:4-5 NIV. "Remain in me as I remain in you. No branch can bear fruit of itself; it must remain in the vine. Neither can you bear fruit unless you remain in me. I am the vine; you are the branches. If you remain in me and I in you, you will bear much fruit; apart from me you can do nothing."

Being connected to Jesus keeps us fresh and green even as we age with new ideas flowing through us bearing fruit. If we fail to stay connected to Him, we cannot bear fruit throughout the length of our life. Many people say, "I'm retired now. I guess I will take it easy," but there is no retirement from Jesus. We can have the very life of Jesus flowing though us at any age, young or old. Stay connected to him.

There is an old song that reminds us that we shall not be moved away from Jesus. We can be determined to plant our feet securely and not be moved away from Jesus throughout our life.

"I shall not be, I shall not be moved.

I shall not be, I shall not be moved,

Just like a tree that's planted by the water, I shall not be move"(Author Unknown).

Chapter 11
Prayer Cloths

The prayer cloth serves as point of contact when you release your faith for healing. It is not something magical but rather a small physical sign of our faith. A person can take the small piece of cloth that has been prayed over and send it to a sick person or pinning it to your own clothes where the pain or sickness is located. Say, "I release my faith now in the Name of Jesus. Body be healed and expect the transition to take place. "I release my faith at this moment in the Name of Jesus." This simple act of faith sets the time for your receiving from the Lord. From the moment you release your faith and deem it to be done, you are not to go back and beg God to do it. Scripture says, "Ask and ye shall receive." That is the now by faith. Not someday maybe. I receive now no matter what I see, hear, or feel in the natural. We receive it in the Spirit first and then it works its way into our physical body. Begin to say positive things from here on out. Be done with saying, "I hurt to saying I am healed in the Name of Jesus."

The prayer cloth is a visible symbol that faith has been released and that healing is on the way. By His stripes we were healed on the cross and to this day by His stripes I am still healed. What do we do between the amen and the there it is? This is a critical time for it is the time the devil brings doubts to our mind. Not only do we need to diligently guard this in between time but do not slip up by what we say. At this point often the devil makes us hurt more than usual or hits us with a more negative doctor's report. Anything to make us doubt God's intention for us will throw us off even more. Do not let anything derail you. Keep the prayer cloth pinned to your clothes over the spot that hurts if this will help remind you that you released your faith and the healing is on the way. Sometimes people will use a larger object as a reminder of the day when they released their faith. Prayer shawls to wrap around them are often the physical symbol that is used to remind us of this transition. Scripture mentioned a type of prayer cloth that was used during Paul's day. Scripture does not refer to them as prayer cloths but rather as handkerchiefs or aprons. Acts 19:11-12 relates how handkerchiefs that Paul had touched were carried to the sick. In modern times the prayer cloths may be prayed over and anointed with oil.

Sometimes a number of people may lay hands on a prayer cloth and then send to the sick person. It can also be a reminder that people are praying as well as a contact point when the person releases his/her own faith.

Chapter 12
The Blood of Jesus

An old song says, "Oh, the blood of Jesus, Oh the blood of Jesus, Oh the blood of Jesus, has never lost its power. Hallelujah, hallelujah, hallelujah for the blood, Hallelujah, hallelujah it has never suffered loss."

The blood of Jesus is not often talked about in church in today's society. It is thought to be deemed passe' but it is still effective today.

Growing up in a church that believed in healing and that it was included in the atonement along with the forgiveness of sins, many songs about the blood come to mind. We were told to "plead the blood of Jesus." What did this mean? I don't think I ever fully grasped what it meant, but I did it to the best of my ability and said out loud, "I plead the blood of Jesus over my body." Looking back at the history of the blood in the Old Testament, the Israelites were faithful to offer a lamb as a sacrifice for sin. It was to be an unblemished animal and this is what John the Baptist referred to when he said, "Behold the Lamb of God" when speaking of Jesus. (John 1:29 KJV).

The Old Testament sacrifices were temporary and had to be repeated. They covered where Jesus cleansed.

When Jesus was on the cross, He said, "It is finished" (John 19:30). Of the sayings of Jesus on the cross none is more important than this one. Jesus came as the final sacrifice for our sins, and his death on the cross was an acceptable one to God. It didn't have to be repeated over and over again down through history. It did not mean Jesus plus one more thing. It meant Jesus, period. Jesus had finished the work God gave him to do. Jesus does not need us to add on something to salvation. Nothing else is needed for salvation. Romans 5:9 says, "Much more then, being now justified by his blood, we shall be saved from wrath through him."

We have been redeemed from the curse of the law. Galatians 3:13 says, "I am redeemed from the curse of the law being made a curse for us: for it is written, cursed is everyone that hangeth on a tree." Jesus has the power to release the grip of the curse through his blood. We are forgiven, we are healed, we have His provision because of what He did on the cross. This provision couldn't happen any other way. People often say, "I don't need a savior. I can save myself, but salvation does not come through a sacrifice of animals no matter how perfect. Hebrews 10:4 says, "for it is not possible for the blood of bulls and goats should take away sins." Hebrews 9:22 tells us, "for without the shedding of blood there is no remission of sins."

We can say with Paul, "I am forgiven. I have redemption through his blood, the forgiveness of sins according to his riches of his grace" (Ephesians 1:7).

What are we to think of the sacrifices of Jesus for our sins and for all the other things made available for us in the atonement? Are we to just go our merry way and say, "Ho hum, that was sure nice of Him to do that for me."

This same blood has the power to release us from the grip of sin. Paul said in Galatians 5:1, "Stand fast in the liberty wherewith Christ hath made us free, and be not entangled again with the yoke of bondage." We have been redeemed from the curse of sin and sickness and poverty. Why are we so often letting the devil hold a curse over us and we become ensnared nd entangled all over again. The blood makes you more than a conqueror.

I Peter 1:18-19 NIV tells us "For you know that it was not with perishable things such as silver or gold that you were redeemed from the empty way of life handed down to you from your ancestors, but with the precious blood of Christ, a lamb without blemish or defect."

I have been moved from the enemy's kingdom in to the kingdom of God. I am able to come close to God. "But now in Christ Jesus you who were once far away have been brought near by the blood of Christ"(Ephesians 2:13 NIV).

Let the blood save you on earth as well as in heaven. All that comes through the blood on earth. Your deliverance comes through the blood of Jesus. Call on the blood for what you need. Plead the blood of Jesus over the works of the enemy. The blood has never lost its power. What will the blood of Jesus do for you? The blood makes you more than a conqueror. "They [we] overcome by the blood of the lamb and the word of [our] testimony" (Rev. 12:11).

Are we failing to overcome life's struggles because we don't realize the power in the blood? Are we tolerating a curse when we have been redeemed from the curse of the law? To be not healed is a curse. It is God's will for you to be healed. Healing was a good thing back in Jesus' day. Healing is a good thing now.

Acts 10:38 says, "God anointed Jesus of Nazareth with the Holy Ghost and with power who went about doing good and healing all that were oppressed of the devil, for God was with him" It is God's will for me to be healed. I decide that healing is the way I'm going to go. I resist sickness and disease. God wants you to resist sickness and disease just as much as you resist sin. Scripture says in James 4:7, "Resist the devil and he will flee from you." Resisting the devil means must be accompanied by submitting to God. We have been redeemed from the curse of the law by the blood of the lamb. I'm done with the curse of sickness that the devil tries to put on me as well as the curse of poverty. Jesus has broken the fetters that chain us by his blood.

"If the blood's applied to my heart, if the blood's applied, someday I'll stand at the great judgment bar, I know that Jesus will not be far, If the blood's applied to my heart, if the blood's applied, there'll be nothing to say, there'll be nothing to pay if the blood's applied" (author unknown).

Chapter 13
The Power of Agreement

"If two of you shall agree on earth as touching anything that they shall ask, it shall be done for them of my Father which is in heaven" (Matthew 18:19).

Praying and declaring the same thing in agreement is powerful. When there is agreement Jesus said it shall be done. Abraham and Sarah agreed. (Hebrews 11:11). Through the power of agreement we can accomplish more.

We can agree with another person as touching a request and expect God to act upon that request. We often think of this scripture that Jesus told His disciples as pertaining just to other people in prayer such as having a prayer partner to lift up requests with, but did you ever think that you should be agreeing with God as well. Did it ever occur to you that God may be ready to give you the desires of your heart but your words are overriding what He wants to do for you because you are not in agreement with Him? He says, "I AM the Lord that healeth you" but you say, "but I'm sick. I'll never get well. I hurt and it doesn't get any better."

That is not agreement with God. He is saying I AM the Lord that healeth you and you are saying, basically, "No, you aren't." We hold God up from performing His promises to us when we disagree with Him and don't even realize what we're doing. Scripture says, "By his stripes we were healed [on the cross] and we say, "but that was a long time ago. I don't feel healed." Our words stop God from bringing it into our body. I Peter 2:24 says, "by his stripes ye are healed." If we were healed then we should be healed now but we often do without because we doubt. We disagree with what God is trying to tell us and think that God is holding out on us when God's telling us, "No good thing will he withhold from them who walk uprightly." Do we believe our symptoms indicating pain or do we believe that He is our healer? Do we say, "Oh, it must not be His will for me." Scripture says that healing was a good thing and Jesus "healed all that were oppressed of the devil" (Acts 10:38).

Do we say, "Well maybe He did then but He may not heal me today. Might not be His will."

Our words are overriding what He wants to do for us and blocking His power to do it. We must be in agreement as touching our desire in prayer. Agreement is powerful in driving out sicknesses and disease in our our body. We can refer to II Corinthians 4:13 says, "I believed; therefore I have spoken." We believe first—

will we put our words in agreement with God first? If He says, "I am the Lord that healeth thee," who are you to dispute His word. Do we believe the God who has the power to drive out sickness and disease in our body but say words to the contrary? How many blessings do we forfeit because we refuse to believe with Him. I think we miss out on a lot of things.

How can we change things for the better? One way is to get our words into alignment with God's. Throughout the day practice speaking something different from what you are used to.   How do you go about aligning your words with His? For example speak aloud non-existent things as if they were already in existence and work toward them in expectation of them coming to pass. Agree with God. "I am the Lord that healeth thee." Speak the promise in faith. Say your Name, "________, I am the Lord that heals you." Add your name to this statement. That is agreeing with God. Say, "Yes, God, I do believe you are healing me now." Leave the if and maybe out of the sentence and never add, "if it be thy will when it comes to healing." The children's bread mentioned in Matthew 15:26-28 was a descriptive phrase that Jesus used to refer to healing. The scripture here states that healing is the children's bread. Jesus was speaking to a Gentile woman who came to Jesus because her child was sick and she needed to receive healing. Although the gospel was not yet open to the Gentiles, He referred to healing as a rightful thing in a child's home. Just as a father provides that necessity—bread-- in a home, Jesus provides healing for us. The Lord wants you healed—any day from any disease and under any circumstances. Be confident of his provision to agree with Him that it shall be done for you. Declare today, "Healing is my portion as a child of God. By the stripes of Jesus my body and mind are completely healed." I agree with God. Stretch your faith by what your words say. Don't sabotage your healing. Sickness is not from God. He wants us healed. Declare, "God's power to heal resides in me." I am nurturing that power by agreeing with God and speaking what He says."

Chapter 14
The Power of Praise

Praise gives us access to God. Sometimes people will say, "I feel that God is a million miles away and my prayers bounce right off of the ceiling." Scriptures tell us to "Draw near to God and he will draw nigh to you" (James 4:8 KJV). How can we draw nigh to God? We can move toward God as we lift our voices in praise to Him. There is power in the act of praise. "Enter his gates with thanksgiving and into his courts with praise; be thankful unto him and bless his name" (Psalm 100:4). We move toward God as we open our mouths to recognize him with our praises.

Psalm 22:3 says that "God inhabits the praises of Israel." God lives in or dwells in the praises of his people. If He dwells in our praise and thanksgiving, we are not only drawing near to Him but He is drawing near to us. If the Lord is dwelling in the middle our praise, He certainly must be mindful of our our thoughts and prayers. Yes, He knows what is on our mind. Scripture says in I John 5:15 "and if we know He hears us in whatever we ask, we know that we have the petitions that we desired of him." Zephaniah 3:17 says, "the Lord thy God is in midst of thee is mighty, he will save he will rejoice over thee with joy, he will rest in his love, he will joy over thee with singing."

Once we enter his courts with praise He is very aware of what is going on in our lives at the moment even when we feel dry as dust inside and feel that our prayers are not getting beyond the ceiling. Not all of our days are filled with sunshine. Sometimes troubles hit and we don't feel the best in the world. This is where scripture tells us to "offer the sacrifice" of praise. What does that mean? We don't always feel like praising the Lord in joyful singing. Sometimes we feel down and sometimes say we are depressed or hurting. This is when it take a sacrifice. Just what is a sacrifice? It is something that is not easy to give. It costs something, it take more effort than what we are willing to put forth, and it is an all uphill thing to do. So why bother? Surely God will understand. Yes, He might understand but he doesn't want the enemy to get the best of us. Praise defeats the enemy that is why there are so many scriptures urging us to praise the Lord and to enter into His courts. We are too often slow to open our mouth and speak the first word. There is a chorus that says, "We bring the sacrifice of praise to the house of the Lord." The subject of the sentence is we. We bring the sacrifice of praise. Too often we are waiting on God to do something when He is waiting on us to make the first move. He has already made the first move by all that Jesus did on the cross. He has provided liberally for our salvation, our healing, our provision as well as other things too numerous to count. Let us enter in. One preacher always opened the service by saying, "Enter in." Do we miss out because we won't enter in? Do we think it is too difficult to offer the sacrifice of praise? Sometimes we don't know where to start or what to say because we haven't been used to doing it. Think of something specific that the Lord has done for you and speak it out. "I praise you Lord for my job. I thank you for my health." It may seem hard to get it out of your mouth. That's the way a sacrifice is.

"We bring the sacrifice of praise into the house of the Lord, we bring the sacrifice of praise into the house of the Lord. And we offer up to you the sacrifice of thanksgiving and we offer up to you the sacrifice of joy."

We bring—we offer.

Praise changes you as well as the atmosphere around you. It lifts the down feeling that settle on you. Someone once said, "You have to make your own sunshine." Praise to God has a way of moving the clouds out and brings the sunshine in.

Romans 4:20 tells us that Abraham grew strong and was empowered by faith as he gave praise and glory to God.

Most versions say, "Abraham staggered not at the promise of God through unbelief; but was strong in faith giving glory to God" or it says he "wavered not."

The praise of Abraham kept him grounded in his faith and caused him to grow stronger. Would that we would use him as a pattern for our own life and let praises to God roll out of our lips.

The devil would like us to fight a needless battle today and when we are a little bit down and a little bit depressed, he continues to nip at our heals and bring us down a little bit more until we talk about how depressed we feel and how bad things are for us. We manufacture our own anxiety and distress when we could have turned things around and nipped things in the bud by offering the sacrifice of praise to God realizing He lives in our praises. He is there whether we feel Him or not. There is a song, "He was there all the time." That means He *is* there all the time. He *is* there in the good days and in the bad days of our life. There is power in the praises of his people. Learn to thank and praise Him in advance for answered prayer. There is power in praise and thanksgiving.

Chapter 15
Imparting
The Life of Jesus

Jesus said, "I am the resurrection and life. He who believes in me though he were dead shall live" (John 11:25). We didn't stay dead in our sins for Ephesians 2:2 says, "and you hath he quickened who were dead in trespasses and sins. Wherein in times past ye walked according to the course of this world." The verse goes on to say, "but God who is rich in mercy, for his great love wherewith he loved us, even when we were dead in sins hath quickened us together with Christ, (by grace ye are saved). "But now in Christ Jesus ye who sometimes were far off are made nigh by the blood of Christ" (verse 23).

Once we have the resurrection life of Jesus into our body we have been changed and no longer have to be defeated by the enemy. Scripture tells us "if any man be in Christ he is a new creature, old things are passed away and all things are become new" (II Corinthians 5:17). We have a tendency to go on living the same old way, but we have been changed by His blood on the cross. What He did for us on the cross is more than the forgiveness of sins. It includes healing for our bodies as well and provision for our earthly needs. Why do we go limping along with sickness and disease and take on ownership for things that tear us down and make us ineffective. The power of God is now in us to drive out sickness and disease. Don't make it your friend where you latch on to it and say, "My diabetes, my fibromyalgia or any number of other things." No, it is time to be done with these things and don't be guilty of tolerating them. If the resurrection life of Jesus is residing in you, would you have pain and sickness? Would Jesus be suffering pain and sickness? Scripture tells us the "power of Jesus was present to heal"—it is in the present tense, not maybe someday. The power of God is at work in our bodies to drive out sickness and disease. We must take our authority over what is plaguing us and speak to the problem with that authority. Say in no uncertain terms, "Pain be gone in the Name of Jesus. I am filled with His resurrection power and sickness cannot stay anymore. Sickness I drive you out now in Jesus' Name. I will not tolerate this disease for another six months. The power of the Lord is present to heal me now, not days or months from now. Luke 5:17 says, "The power of the Lord was present to heal and it is present to heal us today. The resurrection life is renewing and restoring my body. The pain is leaving. The infirmity is leaving. I receive it today. The healing that Jesus provided is flowing through my body like a powerful healing stream into my nerve, cells, and muscles. It is doing the work quietly but surely. I am healed by the blood of the lamb. I have it now. I receive it. I take it. The life of Jesus is all I need. A little chorus we used to sing is, "He's all I need. He's all I need." We don't need Jesus plus something else for our healing. I call forth His healing from my spirit into my physical body. He knows just what we need to make us whole. Why do we think that maybe He doesn't or that He won't do it *for me*. Most people would not deny that He can do it, but they don't know if he will do it for me. The impartation of His resurrection life into our body will not only cure the sin problem but also the sickness and disease problem but we have to believe that He wants us to be healed and living in wellness. What is better than healing? It is to be well as we go through the day. We don't have to let sickness and disease latch on to us. We don't have to invite symptoms into our body. I am healed, I am well in the Name of Jesus.

Chapter 16
When God Answered

Several year ago my shoulder began to hurt for seemingly no reason at all, and I had difficulty getting my arm into my coat sleeve. I had not had an injury to my shoulder and expected it would be well in a few days, but it wasn't. I did everything I knew to do—pain pills, liniment and other arthritic creams, and went to an osteopath, physical therapy and anything else I heard of that I thought might help. I experienced pain every day and nothing helped. The professionals would ask, "What is your pain level" to which I replied that it was pretty high up on the scale of one to ten. I was prayed for repeatedly and used heat on the shoulder about every day. I was anointed with oil and prayed over at church whenever there was a healing line. I was x-rayed and was told I had a tear in the rotator cuff in my shoulder. Week after week went by and I didn't see any improvement, but I didn't know what else to do. The weeks turned into months and I still went to the osteopath on a regular basis. I still went through tubes of pain cream and took prescription pain pills. I tolerated the pain and had learned to live with it, but I still prayed and expected to get better.

One day the osteopath asked me what my pain level was, and I thought about it for a while and answered, "a 3." He didn't believe it but the pain had been gradually subsiding almost to my surprise as well. One day the pain was gone and has never come back to this day. Without fanfare the pain cleared up and the healing took place. I did not require surgery but over a prolonged time I could put my coat on as good with that arm as with the other. I don't know why it took so long but it did. I wish I could say it cleared up rapidly. Sometimes healing takes place quickly and sometime over a period of time. The good news is that it did clear up and healing took place. I think too often we learn to live with pain and tolerate all kinds of inconveniences needlessly. We accept things and invite them to stay longer than we realize that months have gone by and they are still there. Scriptures throughout the Bible tell us that healing is available to us but we do not receive it for one reason or another. We go on year after year allowing sickness and disease to plague us. It is time for us to be free from the chains of sickness and debilitating disease. Satan would like nothing more than to deceive us into thinking that is is maybe not God's will to heal us and that we have to accept things that come on us just as a part of life. There are many statements of faith in scripture that we let slip right by us thinking that they do not apply to us. Hebrews 2:1

says, "Therefore we ought to give the more earnest heed to the things which we have heard, lest at any time we should let them slip."

Too often we don't listen. We don't count what God says in His word very important and we only half hear because we only half listen and we, as a result, forfeit the blessings God has for us. The devil often wins out with his lies because it is his business to "steal, kill, and destroy" (John 10:10). We must learn not to let him put these things on as if they are just to be expected as we go through life. We do not have to take on pain and sickness and disease although we often do. Jesus said, "I come that you might have life and that more abundantly"—it is not life when our bodies are wrecked with pain that nags us day and night. Many time we don't know what to do about situations in our life. James 1: say, "If any man lack wisdom let him ask of the Lord and he will give it liberally." If you have a health problem that you are not seeing any progress being made, ask God for a fresh word about it.

I asked the Lord for a fresh word and expected to hear from him but I didn't immediately. Do we say, I guess He is not going to answer me? Often the answer does not come immediately, the minute we say "Amen" but rather days later there will be a specific thought that flashes through our mind. Do you ever get into a pattern of praying where you ask for the same things over and over and over and you still don't see the slightest hint of an answer? I dare say that is exactly what happens. We have to make some adjustments in our requests. We may need to reframe what we are asking for because we may be asking amiss. James 4:1 says, "and when you do ask you do not receive, because you ask amiss."

We need to reframe our requests if they are not working. A few days later I received a fresh word from the Lord. He impressed this on me. "Do not ask for the same thing over and over again." I could see that this was exactly what I was doing.

The second fresh word came to me a little while later. How often do we disagree with God. When He has already said, "I am the Lord that healeth thee" (Ex. 26:23) we say, "but I still hurt. You must not have healed me." Don't disagree when He says, "by his stripes ye are healed" (I Peter 2:24). We must be open to hearing from God and following what He prompts us to do. We will begin to see results.

Chapter 17
The Strongman

Too many things try to latch on to us—sickness, disease, things that start out small but work their way in over time, a little pain until we can't shake it and it becomes debilitating as time goes by. When we do not rise up to combat the problem, pretty soon we are chained so tightly we can't break loose. Sometimes we become addicted to pain pills to the point of not being able to live without them. We become frustrated because we can't get free no matter what we do.

There is a scripture that tells the parable of what happens to us. It says that no one can enter a strongman's house without tying him up first. Then he can plunder the strong man's house. Jesus refers to Satan as the strong man in the parable and to Himself as the One who enters the house and plunders the place. I John 5:19. Jesus is the One who is stronger than the strong man, and He can bind the strong man, Satan and get control of him.

We must bind the strongman who is Satan and don't let him enter our bodies with sickness and disease. He will bring debilitating pain on us to the point that it incapacitates us. He makes us believe that there is nothing we can do about it. He locks us in chains so tight we cannot get loose, but Jesus said, "Greater is he that is in me than he that is in the world" (I John 4:4). Do we believe that His greater power is within us or do we believe that it is just inevitable that Satan huffs and puffs with all his might to blow our house down or to steal, kill, and destroy anything we will let him take? A well-known verse says, "we wrestle not against flesh and blood but against principalities, against powers, against the rulers of darkness of this world, against spiritual wickedness in high place" (Ephesians 6:12). Another verse tells us more about this adversary. It says, "Your adversary, the devil, prowls around seeking someone to devour" (I Peter 5:8).

Paul said we used to walk "according to the prince of the power of the air, of the spirit that is now working in the sons of disobedience," (Ephesians 2:2). This is why the strong man must first be bound before people can be set free. This is not only true of sin but of sickness. We can be bound with the shackles of sickness to the point where we are paralyzed.

(See: Mark 3:22 and Colossians 1:13).

Satan attempt to set up strongholds against God's people but these strongholds must be brought down with spiritual weapons of the Word of God and the authority that Jesus has delegated to us. The Bible warns us not to let the strongman get an advantage of us for we are not ignorant of his devices. This could be his clever schemes that he uses to trick us into believing his lies.

How do we know we are up to doing anything about Satan. Jesus said, that "he gave us authority to tread on serpents and scorpions and over all the power of the enemy" (Luke 10:19). Another scripture says, "Whatever you bind on earth will be bound in heaven and whatsoever you loose on earth will be loosed in heaven" (Matthew 18:18).

What does this mean to us? We must learn to take action and exercise the authority Jesus has made available. Most of us don't. We need to do more than bind—we must loose something to replace what we have bound. For example, we bound pain and the root cause of that pain. What do we replace it with? We replace pain with healing and wellness. Do not leave any empty space there for the devil to move back with seven more bad things. Scripture gives us an example of what happens. There is one reference, in Luke 11:22 that says "when it [the spirit] arrives, it finds the house unoccupied, swept clean and in order. Then it goes and takes seven other spirits more wicked than itself and they go in and live." He is referring to an impure spirit coming out of a person and it goes through places looking for rest and does not find it. Then it says I will return to the house I left and when it arrives it finds the house unoccupied, swept clean and put in order. Then the spirit takes seven more wicked spirits and moves in. The final stage is worse than what it was at first. Get the devil out and keep him out by filling up the empty space with healing if that is what you need. Get the resurrection power of Jesus into your body and keep the sickness nd disease out. Don't give the devil a foothold. Once the spirit is bound, don't let it stick around. Send it to the pit and tell it not to come back. Once the spirit of infirmity is bound, don't let it linger around and try to regain a foothold. Ephesians 4:27 says, "Leave no room or foothold for the devil." Paul says, "Do not give the devil a foothold—don't make it any easier on him. Send the devil and his demons on their way as soon as you bind them. Send them to the pit and tell them not to come back. Say, "Be gone and mean it." One woman always prayed, "and don't come back for 24 hours." It is better to say, "Don't come back at all. Don't come back period!"

Chapter 18
Speedy Healing

Testimony: My ankle was killing me, and it should have been well weeks ago. I had stepped out of the motorhome and twisted my ankle when we were in Texas. Thinking my ankle would be all right in a couple of days, I didn't have it x-rayed, but when I got back home and back to school my ankle hurt a lot every day by afternoon. I finally listened to my friends who were convinced I had chipped a bone, and had it x-rayed. Nothing showed up in the x-ray, but it still continued to hurt. One day at the Christian school where I was working it was my turn to have hands laid on me and prayed over. They asked me what I wanted prayer for that day and I said my ankle. They gathered around me and laid hands on me and prayed for healing. Nothing visibly happened when they said, "Amen," and I finished my day at work as usual. I didn't think any more about my ankle hurting although it usually did by time to go home. By 10:00 that night it dawned on me that my ankle was not hurting at all. The healing had come speedily and it was healing that lasted and the problem did not come back the next day. Isaiah 58:8 NIV says, "Then your light will break forth like the dawn, and your healing will quickly appear; then your righteousness will go before you and the glory of the Lord will be your rear guard." The King James Version says, "Your health shall spring forth speedily." In this particular case this is exactly what happened.

Other times healing is a much longer process before it happens. I suppose there are many reasons why it happens that way. Do not give up on your healing too quickly. It might come speedily or it might be a longer process. Habakkuk 2:3 says, "for the vision is yet for an appointed time, but at the end it will surely come, it will not tarry."

How long are you willing to wait on a prayer request to be answered? Sometimes I think that in our age of instant technology we are not willing to wait very long. If you have a need for healing, do not give up until you are satisfied with the answer. Don't accept a partial answer and allow people to tell you to just accept things because it not going to be any better now. There are examples of healings in scripture that occurred years after their time to occur, but Jesus made it happen. John 5:5 tells of a man who had been disabled for 38 years sitting by the pool. I imagine this man had about given up after that long a time especially when someone jumped in the water ahead of him when the angel came by to trouble the water. Jesus asked him if he wanted to be well, and the man told him someone always jumped in ahead of him, but Jesus did not leave it at that and walk away. Jesus did something speedily for this man and when Jesus told him to get up and take up his bed and walk, he did it. He had enough hope left that he tried to get into the pool and he had enough hope left to stand on his feet and try to walk. This man didn't even know who had made him well when people asked him. Often we pray about a sickness and time goes by and things don't happen as we expected. Do we get discouraged and say, "I guess He is not going to do it for me and then just learn to accept it? Do we learn to live with it and continue to deny ourselves the results? They may be just around the corner. Although things look slow, our speedily can come in just a short time. There was an old song we used to sing. I Would Not Be Denied.

1. "When pangs of death seized on my soul, unto the Lord I cried; Till Jesus came and made me whole, I would not be denied."

Refrain: "I would not be denied, I would not be denied, Till Jesus came and made me whole, I would not be denied."

2. Old Satan said my Lord was gone and would not hear my prayer, but praise the Lord the work is done and Christ my Lord is here."

Verse two is exactly what happens to us when the devil sneaks around and tell us that Jesus is not going to hear a prayer about our needs of long standing. Friends reinforce that thought and it doesn't take much persuading for us to buy into it. And what tops it off is when a medical professional tells us the same thing. How can we dispute that? When the slightest doubt comes through people telling us that God will withhold good things from us, refer to Psalm 84:11 which tells us that "No good thing will he withhold from them that walk uprightly." Healing for our bodies is a good thing, and we should not be denied because of our own doubts or what people tell us can or cannot happen. Jeremiah 30:17 says, "For I will restore health unto thee, and I will heal thee of thy wounds saith the Lord…"

The Word of God is solid footing for us to stand on in spite of disappointments and delays. A delay is not a denial. The Word of God is "settled in heaven" (Psalm 119:89). The Word of God is more reliable than the opinions of people. Train yourself to take God's Word above all else. When doubts come, be quick to reject them. Say, "No, I am believing what God says because His Word is "settled in heaven."
Verse 3 of this old song speaks of our wrestling with the Lord like Jacob of Old.

3. "As Jacob in the days of old I wrestled with the Lord, and instant with a courage bold I stood upon His word." (Charles P. Jones 1865-1949).

The verse points to our standing on the Word of God above all else no matter what circumstances tell us. Have the courage to stand firm and do not be denied whether the healing comes slowly or speedily.

Chapter 19
Praying in the Spirit

Praying in the Spirit is important as well in our healing experience. Many times we do not know how to pray about something because we can't really pinpoint the problem. Romans 8:26 tells us, "Likewise the Spirit also helpeth our infirmities: for we know not what we should pray for as we ought but the Spirit itself maketh intercession for us with groanings which cannot be uttered." If we try to figure it out on our own, we can miss it totally and not be getting to the source of the problem. Even medical tests may be misdiagnosing the root cause of the problem. The Holy Spirit penetrates the surface and gets to the heart of the problem with sensitivity to what is happening beneath the surface.

The Holy Spirit can determine the will of the Father when praying about something we don't understand. Praying in the Spirit reframes a prayer request from our finite understanding. We may think this is the way it should be but miss it totally. We do not always have to know all the ins and outs of a situation or try to figure it out in detail for how God should solve the problem. Learn to be pliable in the prayer language of the Holy Spirit and let the language flow out of your inner being as it will. It will be saying what needs to be said in an effortless way. Just let it flow out and it will be truly the heart's cry.

Sometimes we are concerned about what we are saying when we pray in an unknown tongue and worry that we are not getting it right; but scripture says we can pray in the Spirit and in the understanding also. Ask the Spirit to show you what you are praying about. It will usually not be a word for word translation of what you are saying but a general impression that you will know you are on the right track.

Praying in the Spirit aligns us to God's will. Where we have been missing it when we pray in English, we come closer to hitting the target. Paul said, "I will pray with the spirit and pray with the understanding also" (I Corinthians 14:15). The New Living Translation says, "I will pray in the spirit and I will also pray in words I understand…" I will cover the need from all angles.

Many of us know that there is an effective way of praying other than in the language we understand, but we don't do it for one reason or another. Maybe praying in tongues has had a stigma about it when we were growing up. We didn't do it in our church, and we were told to stay away from it. We often had the impression that it was from the devil or that it was the Holy Rollers on the other side of the track who did it. It didn't take much convincing to keep us as far away from it as possible because we didn't understand a language that we didn't learn in school. People want to be accepted by others and avoid being criticized. We don't want to look foolish in the eyes of our friends, so rather than being laughed at, we avoid doing anything out of the norm. Another reason we don't pray in the Spirit is because it is time consuming. We often pray a minimum time about things. If God answers, OK, and if He doesn't OK. Must not be His will we say. If we doubt or downright don't believe, we do without. We learn to live with the undesirable circumstance in our life and justify why they are there. We say that is just inevitable. It's the process of aging and we can't do anything about it. We doubt and do without too much of the time. The man at the Pool of Bethesda had Jesus' full attention when Jesus asked him point blank, "Do you want to be well." The man came up with the answer, "Someone always jumps in ahead of me when the angel troubles the water" rather than a clear cut "Yes" Or "No" answer. Praying in the Spirit was made available to us on the day of Pentecost to help us with our many needs and yet we are not taking advantage of His help. The Holy Spirit is our guide. Jesus told His disciples, "When the spirit of truth comes, he will guide you into all the truth…" (John 16:13). He communicates through our prayer language and gets it right the first time. Let us not be so quick to reject things that seem unfamiliar to us because of fear or uncertainty. Let us investigate on our own because others may not have the final answer either. Jesus told his disciples He would send another comforter. John 14:26 tells us what this Comforter will do. "But the Helper, the Holy Spirit whom the Father will send in my Name, He will teach you all things and bring to your remembrance all I said to you." Certainly we would not want to reject the teacher that Jesus said He was sending to us.

In spite of fearfulness and lack of answers, let us enter into a relationship with the Comforter where He can assist us in our struggles with how to pray and what to pray about. He wants us to live a victorious life defeating the devil. God wants us healed and to be done with thing that continually try to plague us and drag us down. Revelation 12:11 tells us that "we overcome by the blood of the lamb and the word of our testimony." Let's move toward that goal by praying in the Spirit about all of our concerns."

Chapter 20
The Healing Power

The healing power is working in you to drive out sickness and disease. We have healing given to us in the form of healing power that goes to work when hands are laid on us, when we speak the Word, when we place an anointed prayer cloth on us or in any number of other delivery systems. The full blown manifestation of healing usually does not occur immediately but rather we get the healing power and it begins to work immediately in our bodies. We keep the switch of faith turned on by having confidence that He is working in the days ahead. Luke 5:17 says, "The power of the Lord was present to heal." It is actively working as long as we adamantly believe. Matthew 10 says, "Heal the sick, raise the dead, cleanse the lepers, drives out demons. Freely you have received, freely give" NLT. We do not concoct the healing power within ourselves. It come from God and we receive it and impart it to others. When others take it by faith, it becomes active to do its work; but you must keep the switch turned on by what we believe and what we say. Some positive statement are necessary. "I believe the power of the Lord is working in me to drive out sickness and disease." At first it may seem that not one thing has changed and the same old aches and pains are in your body. Be persistent to go after the pain by binding it in the Name of Jesus and His power. Command it to be gone in His Name and expect it to go. Make a demand on the promises of God and expect them to produce for you. Speak the Word out loud. "By his stripes I am healed" (I Peter 2:24) is a positive one. Speak it and believe it. Expect it to happen in the days ahead. Do not confess anything negatively but speak what God says in His Word. "By his stripes I am healed" and don't accept anything else. The power of God may work silently in you over a period of time and then one day you realize the pain has gone and you can do things you couldn't do before. It was working in you quietly bringing about the desired result. Don't discount the quiet but thank the Lord in the days when it looks as if nothing at all is happening. Keep in mind that the devil often makes things look worse in the critical time. The pain comes back and the symptoms seem worse. A doctor's report looks worse than it did before. The devil is a master at making you run scared. Panic arises in our heart and fear looms heavy over us. That is the time when we have to stand with our feet firmly anchored on the promise of God and our eyes fixed fully on Jesus. Otherwise we will agree with what the devil is putting into our minds. An old song says, "On Christ the solid rock I stand, all other ground is sinking sand, all other ground is sinking sand." Make a firm decision that you won't step off of the Rock Christ Jesus. The power of God is working in you today to drive out sickness and disease. Sickness and disease cannot stand up to His power and His Name. It may be a battle because it is warfare with the devils tactics but he has already been defeated. Know this from the beginning and don't let anything cause you to waver. At this point the battle is either won or lost. Do you side with God or listen to what people tell you about it and give you advice on what they would do? Do you latch on to the latest pain and worry that this one is going to sink you? Sometimes we think we don't have any choice in the matter, but we can either go with what God says or go with what seems right and the logical advice of others. Scripture says when this happens to "demolish arguments and every pretension that sets itself up against the knowledge of God and we take captive every thought to make it obedient to Christ" (II Corinthians 10:5).

This means getting control over what you think about things. Do not let anything derail your faith. The power of God is working in you to drive out sickness and disease. Even if it takes a while to see it happen, let patience have her perfect work and it will.